Introduction

With so many sources of health information at your fingertips — many of them online — it can be tough to tell fact from fiction, or useful health products and services from those that don't work or aren't safe.

The FTC has created this booklet to help you find reliable sources of information on health topics important to you, whether you're an older consumer or a family member, caregiver, or friend. You can:

- find links to agencies and organizations that care about topics like generic drugs, hormone therapy, caregiving, surgery to improve vision, alternative medicine, hearing aids, Medicare fraud, and medical ID theft;

- learn how to spot misleading and deceptive claims; and

- find out who you can contact to ask questions, enlist help, or speak up if you think a health product or service isn't living up to its promises.

Just remember: Among the best sources of health information is someone you can meet face-to-face. Talk about all of your health-related decisions with your doctors and other trusted health care providers.

If your typical search for health information consists of typing a topic into a search engine, you're not alone. But you're also not guaranteed quality results. The websites that top your search list may not be up-to-date or reliable. Next time, consider starting with sources you can trust. Three great options: MedlinePlus, Healthfinder.gov, and Healthcare.gov.

- MedlinePlus (medlineplus.gov) — Look up a condition or disease at MedlinePlus, and you'll find a page organized to make it easy to find the information you're looking for. Sponsored by the National Library of Medicine — part of the National Institutes of Health (NIH) — the website draws from the Library of Medicine, NIH, other government agencies, and health-related organizations. Other MedlinePlus features include a drug and supplement look-up, an illustrated medical encyclopedia, and current health news headlines and links.

- Healthfinder.gov (healthfinder.gov) — Another one-stop-shop for finding reliable health information online, Healthfinder.gov draws on more than 1,600 government and non-profit organizations to point you to current information. The site — a product of the Office of Disease Prevention and Health Promotion in the Department of Health and Human Services (HHS) — also offers consumer health guides, recent health news by topic, and a directory of health-related organizations.

When it comes to specific websites, the FTC suggests looking for:

- Government websites. Sites ending in .gov, such as the websites for the Centers for Disease Control and Prevention (CDC) at cdc.gov, Centers for Medicare and Medicaid Services at medicare.gov, Food and Drug Administration (FDA) at www.fda.gov/consumer, National Cancer Institute at cancer.gov, National Institute on Aging at www.nia.nih.gov, and National Women's Health Information Center at womenshealth.gov, are produced by agencies of the federal government and generally reflect the most recent research and information.

- University or medical school websites, with web addresses ending in .edu, or sites for well-known, trusted health facilities.

- Websites for not-for-profit groups that focus on research and teaching the public about specific diseases or conditions. These websites typically end in .org, but keep in mind that ".org" doesn't guarantee a site is reputable. Scammers may set up bogus .org sites to rip off consumers.

Table of Contents

Alternative and Complementary Treatments

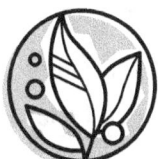 My brother has cancer and is looking into alternative treatments. He has seen ads for a clinic that claims an amazing success rate using unconventional approaches. Should he believe them?

Unconventional treatments for cancer or any other disease can sound tempting when you're hoping for a cure. But researchers don't know how safe or effective many of them are. Many have proven ineffective and even harmful; some haven't undergone rigorous scientific testing at all.

Still, some types of complementary therapy — therapy used with, not instead of, conventional medicine — can be useful. Talk to your doctor about any treatment you're considering. Besides telling you how safe or worthwhile the treatment might be, your doctor can let you know whether it could interfere with other medications and treatments you're getting. And before you believe promises that an alternative or complementary treatment works, ask for a copy of any studies that prove it. Then ask a knowledgeable doctor, pharmacist, or other health care professional to review them. Take testimonials from "real people" with a shaker-full of salt. The testimonials could be embellished or even made up, and those "real people" could be actors, paid to read lines. Learn more from the National Center for Complementary and Alternative Medicine and the National Cancer Institute.

If you're considering treatment at a clinic that's far from home or requires an extended stay, check it out with your doctor. Some clinics offer effective treatments, but others prescribe untested, unapproved "cures" that don't work and may even be dangerous. Sometimes, health care providers who work there are unlicensed or lack basic credentials. For information on a hospital, clinic, or treatment center, contact the health authorities where it's located. If it's in another country, contact that government's health authority to make sure the facility is properly licensed and equipped to handle the procedures involved.

Patients who want to try an experimental treatment should talk to their doctor about how they might enroll in a clinical study. For information on both federally and privately supported clinical trials, visit ClinicalTrials.gov. You also can learn about clinical trials — and when patients may take investigational drugs outside of a trial — at the Office of Special Health Issues on the FDA website.

Who Cares?

National Center for Complementary and Alternative Medicine
nccam.nih.gov
1-888-644-6226
(TTY: 1-866-464-3615)

National Cancer Institute
cancer.gov/cam
1-800-422-6237
(TTY: 1-800-332-8615)

American Cancer Society
cancer.org
1-800-227-2345
(TTY: 1-866-228-4327)

Clinical Trials
ClinicalTrials.gov
clinicaltrials.gov

National Cancer Institute
cancer.gov/clinicaltrials
1-800-422-6237
(TTY: 1-800-332-8615)

FDA
Office of Special Health Issues
www.fda.gov
1-800-216-7331

Internet tip:
Find links to more information on alternative and complementary medicine at MedlinePlus.gov and Healthfinder.gov.

Assisted Living and Nursing Homes

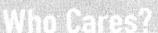

National Clearinghouse
for Long-Term Care
Information
www.longtermcare.gov

Medicare
medicare.gov
1-800-633-4227
(TTY: 1-877-486-2048)

Finding a Facility
Your Area Agency
on Aging
eldercare.gov
1-800-677-1116
(TRS: 1-800-677-1116)

Medicare's Nursing
Home Compare
medicare.gov/nhcompare

American Association
of Homes and Services
for the Aging
aahsa.org

Assisted Living
Federation of America
alfa.org

Senior Housing Locator
seniorhousinglocator.org

American Health
Care Association/
National Center
for Assisted Living
longtermcareliving.com

My dad has lived alone for awhile. Lately, he's had trouble with basic activities like bathing and dressing. I think an assisted-living facility might be a good option for him, but I don't know much about them. Where do I start?

When you realize a parent or loved one needs more help than you can give, you may have to make some big decisions in a short time. Sometimes, with the help of a caregiver, an older person can continue to live at home (for more on caregivers, see page 3). But you may find that an assisted-living facility or nursing home is the best fit. Assisted living allows residents to maintain independence, living in apartments but getting help with daily activities. Nursing homes offer a higher level of care and are best for patients who need regular nursing attention and medical care. For an overview of long-term care options, visit the Medicare website and look for Long-Term Care.

Choosing the right facility takes research. Ask family, friends, and health care providers for recommendations, as well as your local Area Agency on Aging (AAA). Your AAA also should know about other resources for eldercare services and caregiver support in your community. To find and compare Medicare- and Medicaid-certified nursing homes, use Medicare's online Nursing Home Compare tool.

After you narrow your options, visit some facilities to ask questions and get a feel for each place. The sources in the list on the left are good places to start. For example, the Assisted Living Federation of America offers a consumer checklist, and the American Association of Homes and Services for the Aging offers information on what to look for when touring a nursing home.

Once you've chosen a facility, make sure you know its complaint procedure policy and how to have the care plan reviewed in case you have concerns about the level or quality of care.

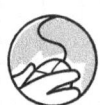

Internet tip:
Get help resolving an issue with a long-term care facility by finding a long-term care ombudsman in your state at ltcombudsman.org.

Hiring Caregivers

My mom needs more care than my siblings and I can manage. To complicate matters, I live in another state. Our mom wants to stay in her home, but we'll need to hire someone to help her. Where should we start?

Caring for a parent, spouse, or someone else you love can be a tough balancing act. Help from home health workers is one way to make it work. But before you hire someone, figure out what services you need, and what services you can afford. For an overview of home health care services available and advice on how to find a qualified and trustworthy home care provider, visit the websites for the National Association for Home Care and Hospice, and the Visiting Nurse Associations of America. To find out about specific services and agencies in a particular community, call your local Area Agency on Aging. You also can use Medicare's Home Health Compare tool at the Medicare website to find Medicare-certified home health care agencies. For the average cost of home health aides and other care in an area, visit the National Clearinghouse for Long-Term Care Information.

Long-distance caregivers may face added challenges. To help, the National Institute on Aging created "So Far Away: Twenty Questions for Long-Distance Caregivers," which you can download or order at the institute's website. Depending on your financial situation, you might consider hiring a local care manager to coordinate your loved one's care. Cost and services vary. Visit the National Association of Professional Geriatric Care Managers website to learn more.

Whether you plan to hire a caregiver or take that job on yourself, other useful resources include the Family Caregiver Alliance and AARP's Caregiving page. For information on caring for someone with Alzheimer's disease, visit the Alzheimer's Disease Education and Referral Center at the website of the National Institute on Aging.

Internet tip:
As you think about hiring someone to care for a loved one, it's a good time to learn how to recognize the signs of elder abuse. Visit the National Center on Elder Abuse at ncea.aoa.gov.

Who Cares?

Your Area Agency on Aging
eldercare.gov
1-800-677-1116
(TRS: 1-800-677-1116)

National Institute on Aging
www.nia.nih.gov
1-800-222-2225
(TTY: 1-800-222-4225)

National Clearinghouse for Long-Term Care Information
www.longtermcare.gov

Family Caregiver Alliance
caregiver.org

AARP
aarp.org/family
1-888-687-2277

Finding a Caregiver

Medicare's Home Health Compare
medicare.gov/HHCompare

National Association for Home Care and Hospice
nahc.org

Visiting Nurse Associations of America
vnaa.org

National Association of Professional Geriatric Care Managers
caremanager.org

Hormone Therapies

MHT and Menopause
National Institute on
Aging
www.nia.nih.gov
1-800-222-2225
(TTY: 1-800-222-4225)

NIH
nih.gov/PHTindex.htm

**National Women's Health
Information Center**
4woman.gov/menopause
1-800-994-9662
(TTY: 1-888-220-5446)

Bio-identical Hormones
FDA
Office of Women's Health
www.fda.gov/womens
1-800-216-7331

**National Center for
Complementary and
Alternative Medicine**
nccam.nih.gov
1-888-644-6226
(TTY: 1-866-464-3615)

Other Hormone Therapy
National Institute on
Aging
www.nia.nih.gov
1-800-222-2225
(TTY: 1-800-222-4225)

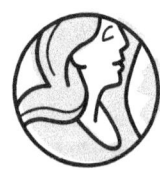

I've been having hot flashes, trouble sleeping, and other symptoms my doctor says are signs of menopause. I've heard menopausal hormone therapy might help, but also that it may be risky. What do I need to know?

Menopause is a natural process that happens as a woman gets older. The amount of estrogen and progesterone her body produces begins to fluctuate and then drop. Menopausal hormone therapy (MHT), once known as hormone replacement therapy, involves taking some of these hormones to keep symptoms of menopause — like hot flashes — under control.

Though MHT has been used for decades and praised for added health benefits like lowering a woman's risk for osteoporosis and colorectal cancer, recent research has uncovered a more complicated picture. Scientists now know it matters when and how long you take MHT. Studies have shown that for some women, using MHT might increase the risk for blood clots, heart attack, stroke, and breast cancer. For more on benefits and risks of MHT, talk to your doctor and visit the NIH website. If you and your doctor decide that menopausal hormone therapy is a good idea, the FDA recommends the smallest dose for the shortest time possible.

You may hear about "natural hormones" or "bio-identical hormones," made by pharmacists and sometimes advertised as a "natural, safer alternative" to MHT. Be cautious. The FDA says there's no credible scientific evidence to support the claims, or the safety or effectiveness of these products. For more information, visit the FDA website.

MHT isn't the only type of hormone therapy. "Anti-aging" hormone therapies aimed at both men and women are based on the same idea — an otherwise healthy person taking a specific hormone that naturally declines with age. Supporters of these hormone therapies claim benefits like improved energy, strength, and immunity, an increase in muscle, and a decrease in fat. Examples include Human Growth Hormone (HGH), melatonin, Dehydroepiandrosterone (DHEA), and testosterone. But while research on these hormones is ongoing, scientists don't yet know what the effects may be. The National Institute on Aging warns that so far, studies haven't proven any influence on the aging process, and each therapy may carry significant risks. To learn more, visit the NIA website and read "Can We Prevent Aging? Tips from the National Institute on Aging."

> **Internet tip:**
> For an overview of menopause, read "Menopause: Time for a Change" at www.nia.nih.gov.

Lasik and Other Vision-Correcting Surgeries

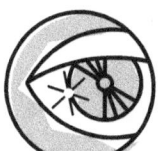 I've worn glasses for 20 years but I'd love to stop. I've heard about Lasik from friends, and I've seen ads that promise 20/20 vision. What do I need to know?

Millions of people have had Lasik eye surgery to correct their vision, and studies show that most people are satisfied with their results. Still, Lasik has risks and possible side effects that can be serious.

Lasik and other vision-correcting surgeries reshape your cornea to refocus light entering your eye. There's no upper age-limit for the surgery, though an age-related eye condition like cataracts can make you a bad candidate for Lasik. But so can factors not tied to your age, like thin corneas. Bad candidates of all ages are much more likely to experience side effects from Lasik, including chronically dry eyes and visual distortions, like double vision or seeing halos around lights. Complications can be temporary, but sometimes they're permanent and debilitating. For more on what you should know about Lasik, visit the FDA website and talk to your ophthalmologist.

As for promises of 20/20 vision — no doctor can make that guarantee. Besides, 20/20 vision still can be flawed vision. And even when your distance vision is corrected, you're likely to need reading glasses when you're over 45. Lasik is just one of several procedures that could improve your vision, and it may not be the best choice for you. Your doctor can help you determine which procedure, if any, is right for you. For an overview, visit the American Academy of Ophthalmology's International Society of Refractive Surgery website. Most insurance companies won't cover these procedures.

Cataract Surgery

My vision is blurry, which makes it hard for me to drive after dark. My doctor says I have cataracts and removing them should fix the problem. I saw an ad for a medical center that says it does risk-free cataract surgery and guarantees clear vision. Should I believe it?

Cataracts, a clouding of the lenses that can lead to blurry vision, are a normal part of aging. Usually, they develop over time and don't have to be dealt with until they interfere with your normal activities. If your doctor says you have a cataract, ask how much you're likely to gain from cataract surgery to replace the cloudy lens and what your risks are. Cataract surgery, done by ophthalmologists in hospitals or eye clinics, is one of the most commonly performed surgeries. Serious complications are rare, but every surgery has risks. To learn more, visit the National Eye Institute.

Internet tip:
For advice on how to find an eye care professional, visit the National Eye Institute at nei.nih.gov/health.

What are living wills and health care proxies? Are they just for people who are terminally ill?

A living will is a document that spells out your wishes for the kind of care you'll receive if you're not in a position to speak for yourself. A "durable power of attorney for health care" is a document that names a "health care proxy" — a person you choose to make health care decisions for you if you can no longer make them. Your proxy can reinforce decisions already spelled out in your living will, or handle situations and decisions your living will doesn't address.

Together, your living will and durable power of attorney for health care are known as "advance directives." For more information about advance directives, visit the websites for National Institute on Aging, the National Hospice and Palliative Care Organization, the National Cancer Institute, or the American Bar Association Commission on Law and Aging, which offers a "Consumer's Tool Kit for Health Care Advance Planning." The kit takes you through questions and issues you may face as you create an advance directive. State laws vary, so be sure your documents and wishes are in line with your state's laws. You may want to consult an attorney. To find resources in your area visit the ABA Commission on Law and Aging's Resources page.

Though advance directives typically deal with end-of-life decisions, you can make the directives — and change them — any time. They also can be used in non-life-or-death situations. For example, people diagnosed with early-stage Alzheimer's disease are encouraged to create advance directives for their care, in addition to legal documents that plan for their finances and estate.

Tell your doctor if you create an advance directive. In fact, talking with your doctor may help you decide whether you want to create a health care directive, and what you want to include.

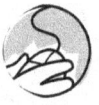

Internet tip:
To find legal services in your area, visit the ABA's findlegalhelp.org. To search for an attorney who specializes in these kinds of issues, check out the National Academy of Elder Law Attorneys at naela.org or the National Elder Law Foundation at nelf.org.

Buying Prescription Drugs Online

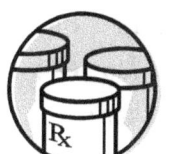

I prefer to shop online if I can save some money. Is there any reason I shouldn't buy prescription drugs or other medical products online?

Shopping online can be a convenient way to look around and compare prices. But when it comes to buying prescription drugs online, be cautious: You could end up with drugs that are fake or include dangerous ingredients. Or, scammers who set up legitimate-looking websites could trick you into giving up personal information that they can use to steal your identity, take your money and send defective drugs, or simply vanish and send nothing at all.

So how do you tell if you're dealing with a reputable pharmacy? The FDA recommends using only websites of U.S.-based pharmacies licensed by a state's board of pharmacy. The National Association of Boards of Pharmacy (NABP) has contact information for your state's board, as well as a list of online pharmacies that have been accredited through its Verified Internet Pharmacy Practice Sites (VIPPS) program (click on Internet Pharmacies). These pharmacies are licensed and meet other NABP criteria. You'll also find a link to sites they don't recommend.

Avoid sites that:

- don't require a prescription

- don't have a licensed pharmacist available to answer your questions

- don't provide their physical business address and phone number

- are based outside the U.S. or aren't licensed by the state board of pharmacy where they are based

A disreputable seller could send drugs that are fake, expired, mislabeled, or the wrong dosage. The drugs could contain dangerous ingredients, or may not be stored or shipped correctly. And if the site is based outside the U.S., there's very little the U.S. government can do if you get ripped off. For more on buying drugs — or other medical products — online, visit the FDA website. And keep in mind that drug prices vary, so you may want to shop around.

For more on saving money with generic drugs, turn to page 9.

Who Cares?

FDA
www.fda.gov/buyonline
1-888-463-6332

Your state board of pharmacy
National Association of Boards of Pharmacy
www.nabp.info

Internet tip: Compare drug prices at different pharmacies online like you would offline, and remember to factor in shipping costs.

Dietary Supplements

I'm thinking about taking dietary supplements to stay healthy. The label says they're all natural and have a lot of benefits. You don't need a prescription to buy them, so they must be safe, right?

Who Cares?

FTC
ftc.gov/health
1-877-382-4357
(TTY: 1-866-653-4261)

FDA
**Center for Food Safety
and Applied Nutrition**
www.cfsan.fda.gov
1-888-463-6332

NIH
**Office of Dietary
Supplements**
ods.od.nih.gov

**National Center for
Complementary and
Alternative Medicine**
nccam.nih.gov
1-888-644-6226
(TTY: 1-866-464-3615)

**National Institute on
Aging**
www.nia.nih.gov
1-800-222-2225
(TTY: 1-800-222-4225)

Healthy Eating
USDA
**Center for Nutrition
Policy and Promotion**
mypyramid.gov
1-888-779-7264

Dietary supplements are products that contain "dietary ingredients" like vitamins, minerals, herbs or other botanicals, amino acids, and enzymes. They range from beneficial to bogus, and you may take them for a host of reasons — to feel healthy, to feel younger, to prevent disease, or just to get more nutrients. Many claim to be "natural."

But just because a supplement is "natural" doesn't mean it's harmless or safe. Some supplements, including herbal products, can be dangerous. For example, there are "natural" supplements linked to serious liver damage and even cancer. And though you can buy dietary supplements off the shelf without a doctor's prescription, some can affect how well your prescription drugs work. Some supplements *do* have proven health benefits: for example, calcium supplements can reduce the risk of osteoporosis. The key is to talk to your doctor — especially if you have a medical condition, take other drugs, or plan to have surgery — before you add a supplement to the mix.

For the latest information on dietary supplements, visit the websites for the National Center for Complementary and Alternative Medicine and the FDA's Center for Food Safety and Applied Nutrition. Dietary supplements don't have to go through the same FDA review for quality, safety, and effectiveness before they're sold that prescription or over-the-counter drug products do. But the FDA requires supplement manufacturers to test the identity, purity, strength, and composition of their products.

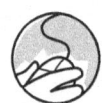

Internet tip:
Look up specific herbs and supplements on the
Drugs and Supplements page at MedlinePlus.gov.

Generic Drugs

My prescription drug costs are pretty high. A friend said she saves money by taking generics. She says they're just as good. Is she right?

Generic drugs are as effective and safe as the brand-name drugs they're based on. They have the same active ingredients and must work the same way as their brand-name counterparts to be approved by the FDA. That means they have the same risks and benefits, too.

Three-quarters of the approved drugs on the market are available in a generic form. The FDA estimates that generic drugs cost 20 percent to 70 percent less than their brand-name counterparts. To see what generic drugs the FDA has approved lately, and for general information on generic drugs, visit the website for the FDA's Office of Generic Drugs.

To find out if there's a generic drug that would work just as well for you as the brand-name drug, talk to your doctor or pharmacist. Say you want the most effective drug at the best price. Each state has a law allowing pharmacists to substitute generic drugs for many brand-name products as long as your doctor doesn't specify that the brand-name drug is required. Contact your state's board of pharmacy to learn more.

Switching Prescriptions

The pharmacist called to say my doctor switched the drug I take for my condition. She says it will save me money, but I'm worried the new drug might not work as well. Can I refuse to switch?

Sometimes, pharmacies and insurance companies get rebates or other incentives when they convince a plan member to switch drugs. But there may be other reasons. If you're uncomfortable about the switch, ask your pharmacist or physician some questions:

- Will the new drug work as well for my condition?

- Are the side effects or risks different?

- Is the dosage the same?

- Is there a business connection between the pharmacist and the drug manufacturer?

- Will the switch save me or my benefit plan money, or cost me more?

If you're still not satisfied, call your state health agency, your state board of pharmacy, or the FDA. They can help you decide if the change makes sense.

Who Cares?

Generic Drugs
FDA
Office of Generic Drugs
www.fda.gov/cder/ogd
1-888-463-6332

Consumer Reports Best Buy Drugs
crbestbuydrugs.org

Drug Questions
FDA
Center for Drug Evaluation and Research
www.fda.gov/cder
1-888-463-6332

Your state board of pharmacy
National Association of Boards of Pharmacy
www.nabp.info

Your state health agency
FDA
www.fda.gov/oca/sthealth.htm
1-888-463-6332

Internet tip: Look up information on specific generic and brand-name drugs on the Drugs and Supplements page at MedlinePlus.gov.

At–Home Genetic Tests

Who Cares?

National Library of Medicine Genetics Home Reference
ghr.nlm.nih.gov/handbook/testing
1-888-346-3656
(TTY: 1-800-735-2258)

FTC
ftc.gov/health
1-877-382-4357
(TTY: 1-866-653-4261)

National Human Genome Research Institute
genome.gov

CDC
National Office of Public Health Genomics
cdc.gov/genomics

National Cancer Institute
cancer.gov/cancertopics
1-800-422-6237
(TTY: 1-800-332-8615)

FDA
Center for Devices and Radiological Health
www.fda.gov/cdrh
1-888-463-6332

I'm thinking of ordering a DNA test that I can take at home. I just need to swab the inside of my cheek and send in the sample. Is this a gimmick, or do these tests really work?

Genetic tests look for signs in your DNA that you're more likely to have particular diseases or disorders during your lifetime. Not long ago, genetic testing was done only when requested by doctors or other health care providers. But recently, "do-it-yourself" tests have become more popular. Typically, you send a blood sample drawn at a clinic or a swab of the inside of your cheek to a laboratory to analyze. Some companies ask you to fill out a questionnaire, too. But according to the FDA and CDC, many genetic tests on the market have no scientific validity, and others may give you results that are vague or meaningful only with a full medical evaluation.

Still, some companies say their tests will tell you how likely you are to get a specific disease — such as heart disease, diabetes, cancer, or Alzheimer's. Others claim they can tell you what diseases you're most likely to get, or how your body might respond to specific treatments. Some go so far as to suggest specific treatments, foods, or nutritional supplements, and offer a customized mix of supplements — usually at an exorbitant price.

Most of the time, your likelihood of developing a disease depends on a number of factors, including diet, lifestyle, and what you're exposed to. Even an accurate genetic test is telling you about only one factor. No standards govern the reliability or quality of at-home genetic tests. The FDA and CDC recommend that genetic tests be done in a specialized laboratory and that a doctor or counselor with specialized training interpret the results.

If you decide to use an at-home genetic test, talk to your doctor or health care provider about which test might be best, and discuss the results with your provider afterward. Check to see how the company will protect your personal information.

Internet tip:
If you decide to use an at-home genetic test, read the privacy policy posted online. It should tell you how the company protects your information.

Vision Prescription Portability

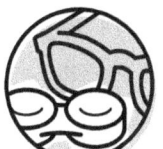

My eye doctor just told me my prescription has changed. I'd like to shop around for new glasses, but the doctor didn't give me a copy of my new prescription. What can I do?

Ask for it. Your eye care provider should always give you a copy of your prescription, even if you don't ask for it. The same is true for contact lens prescriptions. It's the law. The FTC enforces the contact lens and eyeglass rules, which give you the right to your prescriptions so you can buy your eyewear where you like — from an eye care provider, such as an optometrist, ophthalmologist, or dispensing optician, or from a seller, like a specialty shop, large wholesale store, or online retailer.

Expect to get your eyeglass prescription at the end of your eye exam, and your contact lens prescription after your fitting. Even if you don't need your prescription yet, you can file it with your other medical records. If an eye care provider refuses to give you your prescription, report it to the FTC.

If you'll be shopping for contact lenses, remember that all lenses — even cosmetic ones that change the appearance of your eye but don't correct your vision — require a prescription. If lenses don't fit correctly, or aren't used and cared for properly, they can cause problems like corneal ulcers, which can lead to blindness, conjunctivitis (pink eye), or scratches and sores on your cornea. Avoid any seller who doesn't require a prescription. For more on buying contact lenses, visit the FDA's website. To learn more about taking care of your eyes, visit the American Academy of Ophthalmology's EyeCare America website, and the website for the American Optometric Association.

Who Cares?

FTC
ftc.gov/health
1-877-382-4357
(TTY: 1-866-653-4261)

American Academy of Ophthalmology
eyecareamerica.org
1-877-887-6327

American Optometric Association
aoa.org
1-800-365-2219

Contact Lenses
FDA
Center for Devices and Radiological Health
www.fda.gov/cdrh
1-888-463-6332

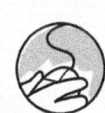

Internet tip:

If you plan to buy your eyewear from an online retailer, do your research. Order only from companies you're familiar with, and find out what happens if there's a problem with your order.

Hearing Aids

Who Cares?

National Institute on Deafness and Other Communication Disorders
www.nidcd.nih.gov
1-800-241-1044
(TTY: 1-800-241-1055)

American Academy of Audiology
audiology.org
1-800-222-2336

Academy of Doctors of Audiology
audiologist.org
1-866-493-5544

American Academy of Otolaryngology
entnet.org

American Speech-Language-Hearing Association
asha.org

Better Hearing Institute
betterhearing.org
1-800-327-9355

AARP
aarp.org
1-888-687-2277

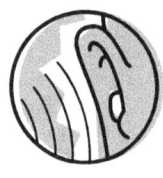

I often ask people around me to repeat what they say, and I need to turn up the volume on my TV. I think I might need a hearing aid. I've seen ads for hearing aid dealers who guarantee satisfaction. What else do I need to know?

Almost 40 million Americans deal with hearing loss. But not all of them can be helped by a hearing aid. That's why it's a good idea to visit an otolaryngologist, a physician who specializes in the ear, nose, and throat, before you buy. It's possible your hearing loss is caused by a medical condition, and treating the condition would improve your hearing. Or, you might find that you have a type of hearing loss that an aid won't help. A medical evaluation is so important that the FDA requires hearing aid sellers to tell you about your need for one before you buy. If you decide not to have a medical evaluation, you must sign a waiver.

If your doctor thinks a hearing aid could help you, you'll need to get a hearing test and fitting by a licensed hearing health professional, like a qualified audiologist. Look for someone who offers products from several manufacturers so you can find the best aid for your needs. Then check out the sellers with your local Better Business Bureau (BBB), consumer protection agency, or state Attorney General (AG). Find out whether dispensers and audiologists need to be licensed or certified by your state, and what other protections you have under state law.

When you shop for an aid, ask if there's a trial period so you can test it. Most states require one, and even in states that don't, most audiologists will offer it. Be sure to find out what fees are refundable if you return the aid during the trial period, and get the details about guarantees and warranties. It's important to get this information in writing. Check whether the price quoted includes testing and other services, as well as the aid. If you buy an aid, but believe the seller isn't living up to a guarantee, file a complaint with your state AG, BBB, or the FTC.

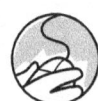

Internet tip:
Buying a hearing aid online can be risky. An aid needs to be custom fitted and tested to be sure it's working properly.

Personal Emergency Response Systems

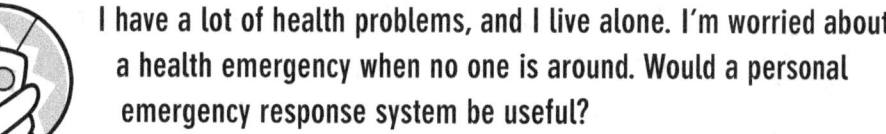

I have a lot of health problems, and I live alone. I'm worried about a health emergency when no one is around. Would a personal emergency response system be useful?

Personal Emergency Response Systems (PERS), also known as Medical Emergency Response Systems, let you call for help in an emergency by pushing a button. A PERS has three components: a small radio transmitter, a console connected to your telephone, and an emergency response center that monitors calls.

Transmitters are light-weight, battery-powered devices. You can wear one around your neck, on a wrist band, on a belt, or in your pocket. When you need help, you press the transmitter's help button, which sends a signal to the console. The console automatically dials one or more emergency telephone numbers. Most PERS are programmed to telephone an emergency response center. The center will try to find out the nature of your emergency. They also may review your medical history and check who should be notified.

You can purchase, rent, or lease a PERS. Keep in mind that Medicare, Medicaid, and most insurance companies typically don't pay for the equipment, and the few that pay require a doctor's recommendation. Some hospitals and social service agencies may subsidize the device for low-income users. If you buy a PERS, expect to pay an installation fee and a monthly monitoring charge. Rentals are available through national manufacturers, local distributors, hospitals, and social service agencies, and fees often include the monitoring service. Read the contract carefully before you sign, and make note of extra charges, like cancellation fees. For more on how to shop for a PERS, visit the FTC website.

Your local Area Agency on Aging may be able to tell you what systems are available in your area. See if friends, neighbors, or relatives have recommendations. When you have a list of agencies you're considering, check with your local consumer protection agency, state Attorney General, and Better Business Bureau to see if any complaints have been filed against them. Questions you can ask a PERS company include:

- Is the monitoring center open 24/7? What kind of training do staff receive?

- What's the average response time, and who gets alerted?

- Will I be able to use the same system with other response centers if I move? What if I move to another city or state?

- What's your repair policy? What happens if I need a replacement?

- What are the initial costs? What costs are ongoing? What kind of services and features will I get?

Who Cares?

FTC
ftc.gov/health
1-877-382-4357
(TTY: 1-866-653-4261)

Your Area Agency on Aging
eldercare.gov
1-800-677-1116
(TRS: 1-800-677-1116)

Checking Out a PERS Company
Better Business Bureau
bbb.org

Your state Attorney General
naag.org

Your local consumer protection agency
consumeraction.gov/state.shtml

Internet tip: Your options when it comes to PERS may depend on where you live. Try looking up your local Area Agency on Aging at eldercare.gov, and ask them about your options.

Weight Loss Promises

Who Cares?

Weight Loss Claims
FTC
ftc.gov/health
1-800-382-4357
(TTY: 1-866-653-4261)

Health and Nutrition
National Institute of
Diabetes and Digestive
and Kidney Diseases
Weight-control
Information Network
win.niddk.nih.gov
1-877-946-4627

CDC
Division of Nutrition,
Physical Activity and
Obesity
cdc.gov/nccdphp/dnpa
1-800-311-3435

USDA
Center for Nutrition
Policy and Promotion
mypyramid.gov
1-888-779-7264

FDA
www.fda.gov/loseweight
1-888-463-6332

American Dietetic
Association
eatright.org
1-800-877-1600

I've always had trouble keeping my weight down. I've heard about a pill that helps you lose weight — and you don't have to stop eating the foods you love or start exercising all the time. Could this really work?

Getting to a healthy weight now can lower your risk for all kinds of diseases later. It's never too late to start. But pills, patches, and creams promising quick, easy, and lasting weight loss aren't worth the money or the risk. As promising as claims may sound, doctors, dieticians, and other experts agree that the best way to lose weight — and keep it off — is to eat fewer calories and increase your activity so you burn more energy. There's nothing you can wear or apply to your skin that will cause you to lose weight. While there is a weight loss pill approved by the FDA for prescription and over-the-counter use by people who are overweight, it's designed to be used along with exercise and a reduced-calorie, low-fat diet. To learn more, visit the FDA website.

When you see a weight loss product, read the claims. Be skeptical when you see:

"Lose weight without diet or exercise!"

"Lose weight permanently!"

"Lose 30 pounds in 30 days!"

"Everybody will lose weight!"

The reality is that the quicker you lose the weight, the more likely you'll gain it back. Experts recommend a goal of losing about a pound or two a week. Even if a product promising lightning-fast weight loss causes you to lose weight, it also could be hurting your health. To learn more about false weight loss claims, visit the FTC website.

The federal government has many resources on safe and effective ways people can lose weight, including those listed on the left.

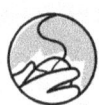

Internet tip:
To check if you're at a healthy weight, calculate your body mass index (BMI) — a measure of weight adjusted for your height — at the CDC website.

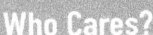

Medical ID Theft

What is medical ID theft, and how is it different from any other identity theft?

Medical identity theft happens when someone steals your personal information and uses it to commit health care fraud. Medical ID thieves may use your identity to get treatment — even surgery — or to bilk insurers by making fake claims. Repairing damage to your good name and credit record can be difficult enough, but medical ID theft can have other serious consequences. If a scammer gets treatment in your name, that person's health problems could become a part of your medical record. It could affect your ability to get medical care and insurance benefits, and could even affect decisions made by doctors treating you later on. The scammer's unpaid medical debts also could end up on your credit report.

You can catch medical identity theft early on. First, read every "Explanation of Benefits" statement you get from your health insurer. Follow up on any item you don't recognize. At least once a year, ask the health insurers you've been involved with for a list of the benefits they paid in your name. Finally, make it a regular practice to check your credit reports. You're entitled to a free report from each of the three nationwide companies every 12 months. You can order your free credit report at AnnualCreditReport.com. For more about your rights, visit the FTC website.

If you think you may be a victim of medical identity theft, ask your health care provider or hospital for your medical records. You have a right to get copies of your current medical files from each health care provider, though you may have to pay for them. You also have a right to have inaccurate or incomplete information removed. Learn more about your rights under federal law at the Department of Health and Human Services (HHS) website. If a health care provider refuses, you can file a complaint with the HHS Office of Civil Rights. Your state provides rights, too. You can look up your state's laws online at the Georgetown University Center on Medical Rights and Privacy. Many hospitals have ombudsmen or patient advocates who also can help.

For more information on protecting personal information, visit the FTC website.

Who Cares?

FTC
ftc.gov/credit
ftc.gov/idtheft
1-877-382-4357
(TTY: 1-866-653-4261)

Health Insurance Portability and Accountability Act (HIPAA)
Department of Health and Human Services
hhs.gov/ocr/hipaa
1-800-368-1019
(TTY: 1-800-537-7697)

Getting Your Free Credit Report
AnnualCreditReport.com
annualcreditreport.com
1-877-322-8228

Your State's Laws
Georgetown University Center on Medical Rights and Privacy
ihcrp.georgetown.edu/privacy/records.html

Your state Attorney General
naag.org

Internet tip:
You don't need to wait until your wallet is stolen to get your free credit report from each of the consumer reporting companies. You're entitled to a free report from each one every 12 months at annualcreditreport.com.

Who Cares?

Medicare
medicare.gov
1-800-633-4227
(TTY: 1-877-486-2048)

**Your State Health
Insurance Assistance
Program (SHIP)**
medicare.gov
1-800-633-4227
(TTY: 1-877-486-2048)

FTC
ftc.gov/idtheft
1-877-438-4338
(TTY: 1-866-653-4261)

Reporting Fraud
**Department of Health
and Human Services
Office of Inspector
General**
oig.hhs.gov/hotline.html
1-800-447-8477
(TTY: 1-800-377-4950)

**Your Senior Medicare
Patrol**
smpresource.org
1-877-808-2468

**Finding a Free or
Low-cost Clinic**
**Health Resources and
Services Administration**
findahealthcenter.hrsa.gov
1-888-275-4772
(TTY: 1-877-489-4772)

**Partnership for
Prescription Assistance
Free Clinic Finder**
pparx.org/
FreeClinicFinder.php
1-888-477-2669

Last month I visited a clinic giving free checkups to people who have Medicare. When I looked at my Medicare notice today, I saw charges I didn't recognize. Did they charge me after all?

Medicare fraud happens when someone intentionally uses your Medicare number to bill Medicare for services or equipment you didn't get or didn't need. The culprit could be a care provider, a scam artist who got your patient identification number through a sham clinic, or an employee with access to your records. And it costs the government billions of dollars each year.

What can you do? Check your monthly Medicare statements. If you aren't sure about a charge, first call the person or company who provided the service. Most errors are honest mistakes. If you still aren't sure about a charge, call the Customer Service number on your statement. Or call your State Health Insurance Assistance Program (SHIP). The number is on the Medicare website. If you believe the charge may be fraudulent, contact your local Senior Medicare Patrol or report it to the Department of Health and Human Services' Office of Inspector General.

Protect your Medicare number by carrying it and giving it out only when you need to. For general information on protecting your personal information, visit the FTC.

Be skeptical of clinics or providers who advertise free services specifically for Medicare patients. If you need to find a federally-funded health center that is free or low-cost, visit the Health Resources and Services Administration or use the Partnership for Prescription Assistance's Free Clinic Finder. If you don't have a computer at home, visit your local library.

Internet tip:
Have questions about Medicare?
Go to Medicare.gov.

Medicare Part D Plans

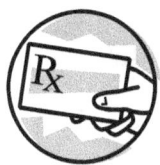 **I'm getting calls about switching to a new Medicare prescription drug plan. The caller says the plan will save me money. He said I could enroll on the phone. How do I know what I'm getting?**

Medicare Part D plans are prescription drug plans that work like insurance, and they're open to anyone with Medicare. The right plan may help control your future drugs costs and may even lower your current costs.

Each Part D plan is different — each can cover different drugs or be available only in a certain area. Medicare doesn't operate the plans; it simply approves insurance companies or other private companies to do that job. But the providers have to follow Medicare rules that limit how they promote their plans. Unfortunately, some plan representatives occasionally break the rules and use high-pressure sales tactics and false promises to try to enroll you in a plan that may not cover the drugs you take. Or, scammers may pretend to be Part D providers trying to get your personal information — such as your Medicare number — to commit ID theft.

It's important to know the rules and do business only with providers that follow them. People who represent Medicare drug plans can't send you emails you didn't ask for or show up at your house uninvited. They can't charge you a fee to enroll or ask you to pay by phone or online. They must send a bill. They can call to tell you about a plan if you're not on the National Do Not Call Registry, but they can't sign you up unless you call them. For more on Part D solicitations and how to protect yourself, visit the FTC website. Report rule-breakers to the Medicare Drug Integrity Contractors (MEDICs) program.

Learn more about Medicare Part D and compare plans available in your area at Medicare.gov. Your State Health Insurance Assistance Program (SHIP) also can point you to local resources that offer free customized advice. Look up your SHIP at the Medicare website.

Internet tip: To find and compare Part D plans, use the Medicare Prescription Drug Plan Finder at Medicare.gov.

Miracle Cures

I saw an ad that said, "CURE YOUR ARTHRITIS WITHOUT DRUGS USING THIS ALL-NATURAL, GOVERNMENT-APPROVED REMEDY." A natural remedy appeals to me, but poison ivy is natural, too. Seems like some products promise more than they can deliver. How can I tell if this one really works?

Miracle products claim to cure serious conditions — often conditions that science has no cure for, like arthritis, diabetes, Alzheimer's disease, multiple sclerosis, cancer, and HIV-AIDS. Some products even claim to be a "cure-all" for several diseases and a host of symptoms. Often, the ads claim the products come with money-back guarantees. Unfortunately, these products, devices, and treatments often are unproven and useless, making promises they can't fulfill.

The reality is that phony miracle products can have dangerous interactions with medicines you're already taking. They also might cause you to delay or stop medical treatment for your condition, even when proven treatments are available from your physician. And a money-back guarantee may be meaningless. It can indicate that a scammer is planning to take your money and close up shop.

Products that claim to do it all often do none of it. So even though you want to believe them, be skeptical, and avoid products that:

- claim to cure incurable conditions

- make extraordinary promises like "shrinks tumors"

- promise a long list of benefits, including "treats rheumatism, arthritis, infections, prostate problems, ulcers, cancer, baldness, and more!"

- are promoted with phrases like "scientific breakthrough," "ancient remedy," or "miraculous cure," or scientific-sounding terms like "thermogenesis"

Always talk to your doctor, pharmacist, other healthcare professional, or public health organizations before you try any new treatment.

Prescription Assistance Programs

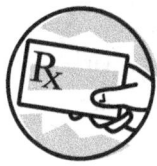

I need help paying for my prescriptions. I heard an ad on the radio for a number to call to see if you qualify for free prescriptions. When I called, they said I was eligible, but I had to pay a pretty big fee. Is this a scam?

Prescription assistance programs, or PAPs, enable people who can't afford to pay for their medications to get them for free or a reduced price. Typically, the programs are sponsored by prescription drug companies or your state. Your financial situation, the cost of the drugs, and whether you have other prescription drug coverage help determine whether you qualify for a prescription assistance program.

Emails, ads, and websites for companies that guarantee free or low-cost prescription drugs for a hefty fee upfront are scams. You are paying for information and applications that are available for free. And even if the company applies to legitimate programs on your behalf, you still may be turned down for the prescription assistance program.

If you think you may be eligible for free or low-cost prescription drugs, you don't have to pay to find out. Ask your physician or pharmacist, or visit one of the websites on this page. For example, the Partnership for Prescription Assistance (PPA) helps consumers find prescription drug coverage. After you enter the prescription medicines you take and answer several questions about your prescription and financial situation, the site directs you to programs you may be eligible for. You can apply online, or you can ask your health care provider to do it for you. Either way, health care providers usually need to approve applications. If you need information on free or low-cost providers and clinics in your area, visit the federal Health Resources and Services Administration or use PPA's Free Clinic Finder. While all Medicare patients can search for Medicare Part D plans on the internet, those who may qualify for extra help can find more information from the Social Security Administration.

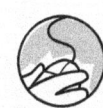

Internet tip:
If you don't have a computer at home, ask a trusted family member or friend if they can help, and talk to your doctor.

How to File a Complaint

The key to an effective consumer complaint is knowing where — and when — to file it. Have you given the company a chance to fix the problem? Often, a brief letter explaining what happened and what you hope the company will do can make a difference. But if the company won't right a wrong, or if you suspect fraud, it's time to file a complaint.

If your complaint is about a health product or service, you may want to contact one of the organizations below. But first, make sure you have important information on hand, like the name and address of the company. Filing a complaint won't guarantee your problem gets fixed, but it can help build a case against a business later. For example, while the FTC can't help individual consumers, its complaint database is a resource for law enforcement agencies all over the U.S. and abroad.

To report deceptive business practices or other types of consumer fraud:

- **FTC** — Go to ftc.gov/complaint, or call 1-877-382-4357 (TTY: 1-866-653-4261).

- Your state **Attorney General** — Find a list of state AGs at naag.org.

- **Better Business Bureau** — File a complaint about a business, website, or non-profit or charitable organization at complaint.bbb.org.

- Your local **consumer protection office** — Find an office near you at consumeraction.gov. Look under "Where to File a Complaint."

To report problems with a medication or medical device:

- **FDA** — Find out where your complaint should go at www.fda.gov/opacom/backgrounders/problem.html.

To report scams and suspicious activity involving Medicare:

- **HHS Office of Inspector General** (OIG) — Call the OIG's fraud hotline at 1-800-447-8477 (TTY: 1-800-377-4950).

- **FTC** — Visit ftc.gov/complaint, or call 1-877-382-4357 (TTY: 1-866-653-4261).

To report fraud or abuse related to a Medicare Part D prescription drug plan:

- **Medicare Drug Integrity Contractors** (MEDICs) — Call 1-877-772-3379.

For help with a complaint about a long-term care facility:

- Your **state long-term care ombudsman** — Find an ombudsman with the Ombudsman Locator at ltcombudsman.org.

To report suspected elder abuse, neglect, or exploitation:

- **National Center on Elder Abuse** — Visit ncea.aoa.gov, or call 1-800-677-1116.

October 2008

Websites and phone numbers are current at press time.

www.ingramcontent.com/pod-product-compliance
Lightning Source LLC
Chambersburg PA
CBHW080809290526
45790CB00008B/3631